MW00974278

"When v _____ hos-
pital, my _____ :ome
with an ii _____ *action*
Book is the comprehensive manual we didn't have. It
is a must-read, especially for new fathers. Sherry Kelly
hits a homerun as she walks new fathers and mothers
through the excitement and challenges of welcoming a
new member into the family."

—Clarke Stroud,
University Vice President for Student Affairs and Dean
of Students, University of Oklahoma, Norman, Oklahoma

"I would highly recommend this book to any new
parent. Mrs. Kelly gives accurate and concise advice
throughout her book. It is perfect for the already sleep-
deprived and time-crunched new mom or dad. With
wisdom and humor, this book truly celebrates the miracle of watching a child grow."

—Kimberly Edgmon, MD, FAAP

"Sherry Kelly has always been an inspiration to me and
I have always admired her parenting skills. Many times
I have asked her advice in raising my four children."

—Verna Scott, LPN,
Retired

"I recommend this book to everyone–parent or not.
The positive influence and advice Sherry Kelly has is
amazing!"

—Troy Chavez,
Dad of an active nineteen-month-old

"If anyone can write the perfect book on this subject, it is Sherry Kelly! Her advice, influence, and support are endless and help me every day! Thank you!"

—Amy Pitzer-Chavez,
Mom of an energetic toddler

"As a gifted educator, Sherry Kelly is highly qualified to help young families answer the multitude of questions that come with the addition of a new baby. Her understanding of child development and creative teaching skills allow her to provide well-qualified advice to parents as they face the rewards and difficulties of raising exceptional children."

—Holli Sills, Healthy Families
Support Worker 1997–2000

"Sherry Kelly's *Instruction Book* demystifies for first-time parents the experience of caring for a new baby. Bridging a gap between pregnancy and toddler parenting publications, Kelly shares practical wisdom gained from over ten years of serving as a parent educator in an easy to read, step-by-step format. Inexperienced mothers and fathers will gain both the knowledge and confidence needed to nurture their newborn in his/her formative first year of life. An ideal baby gift, and a must have addition for the bookshelves of all parents."

—Robin Stroud,
Assistant to the Executive Vice President
and Vice President for Administration and
Finance, University of Oklahoma

Your New Baby's
INSTRUCTION BOOK

Michelle —
I haven't read this book yet — but Sherry is a friend of mine and I know it will be helpful! Hope you enjoy! I still can't quite get over having found you again after all of these years. You are a kindred spirit of mine — you actually taught me something about.

XO, dana
4/10

SHERRY KELLY

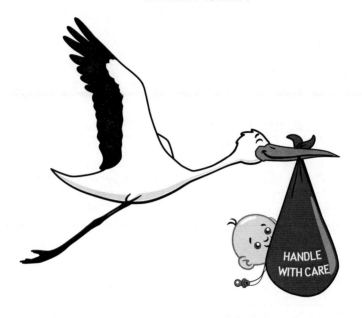

Your New **Baby's**
INSTRUCTION
BOOK

Tate Publishing & *Enterprises*

Your New Baby's Instruction Book
Copyright © 2008 by Sherry Kelly. All rights reserved.

No part of this publication may be reproduced, stored in a retrieval system or transmitted in any way by any means, electronic, mechanical, photocopy, recording or otherwise without the prior permission of the author except as provided by USA copyright law.

Scripture quotation is taken from the Holy Bible Contemporary English Version. Copyright © 1995, American Bible Society.

This book is designed to provide accurate and authoritative information with regard to the subject matter covered. This information is given with the understanding that neither the author nor Tate Publishing, LLC is engaged in rendering legal, professional advice. Since the details of your situation are fact dependent, you should additionally seek the services of a competent professional.

The opinions expressed by the author are not necessarily those of Tate Publishing, LLC.

Published by Tate Publishing & Enterprises, LLC
127 E. Trade Center Terrace | Mustang, Oklahoma 73064 USA
1.888.361.9473 | www.tatepublishing.com

Tate Publishing is committed to excellence in the publishing industry. The company reflects the philosophy established by the founders, based on Psalm 68:11,
"The Lord gave the word and great was the company of those who published it."

Book design copyright © 2008 by Tate Publishing, LLC. All rights reserved.
Cover design by Kandi Evans
Interior design by Kellie Southerland

Published in the United States of America

ISBN: 978-1-60604-692-0
1. Family & Relationships: Child Development
2. Christian Living: Relationships: Parenting
08.12.22

To Kelli, Chad, and Piper
Who came without instructions
And in memory of my parents who
parented with unconditional love

NEW PARENTS MANUAL

Welcome to the world of parenting!
Congratulations on the arrival of your new baby!

TABLE OF CONTENTS

FOREWORD

What a wonderful gift this book is for new parents. It is the fruit of years of experience and is coated with love for children. Sherry Kelly and I met when she applied for a job with the Oklahoma State University Cooperative Extension as a parent educator, a job designed to provide new parents with information and support during pregnancy and continuing throughout the first five years of their lives as a family.

Before becoming a parent educator, Sherry studied child development in college, was a home day-care provider, was foster mom to 15 children, taught postnatal classes in local hospitals, and with her husband, raised their own three children.

Even with all of this knowledge and experience, Sherry was open to learning new skills that would benefit her clients. These achievements included becoming a certified breastfeeding educator through the lactation consultant services affiliated with the

Oklahoma City Mercy Health Center, becoming a certified child and parenting assistant through the Oklahoma Family Resource Coalition (OFRC), and passing certification to properly administer and interpret the DENVER II child development screening tool.

Many times Sherry encountered an issue of importance to her families and could not find the specific topic available. In order to meet the needs of her clients, Sherry researched and wrote several articles that became valuable contributions to our curriculum. These additions to the parent education curriculum were approved by a Child Development Specialist at OSU and were greatly appreciated by her peers as well as her client families.

In the ten years Sherry was employed by the OSU Extension Service as a parent educator, her job title changed along with the name of the program. The program took on the new title of Healthy Families and at that time she became certified as a family support worker. While Sherry was active in the program it received several awards for excellence.

Sherry set the precedent of nurturing a family the entire five years and was instrumental in acknowledging and celebrating the graduations of numerous families from the program. She was available as a mentor and advocate when appropriate and assisted families in ways beyond providing the weekly home visit.

This book is an excellent introduction to the wisdom needed for successful parenting and having this resource so readily available will be a source of comfort and assurance to the reader.

—Carole L. Garner, MS,
Parent Education Program Manager, Retired

PRELIMINARY INSTRUCTIONS

If you are reading this during your pregnancy, you have a great head start on the knowledge needed to parent a newborn. This will be to your advantage and help you to be better prepared when your baby arrives. I would also urge you to get a good book on pregnancy to help guide you along the best path during your baby's wonderful and consequential journey into life.

If perchance you are reading this before your baby's birth, consider banking or donating the cord blood. Harvesting cord blood is simple and painless. The cord blood contains stem cells which can be used to treat a growing number of diseases and disorders. It is good to be prepared for this before you go into labor, so ask your doctor about making the arrangements in advance.[1]

This book takes up where pregnancy ends–with the birth of your own little miracle of life!

The information in *Your New Baby's Instruction Book*

covers the basics for a successful first year with your new little son or daughter. It is beneficial to all parents from young, first-time moms and/or dads to the more mature experienced parents. If you have adopted your new addition, this book is meant for you as well.

As a parent educator, I often commented about the need for parent education because "babies didn't come with an instruction book." Parenting is one of the—if not *the*—most important jobs we will ever have. After all, the world's future depends on today's children. Yet it is the job for which we are probably the least prepared. For the most part, parenthood results in "on the job training." We learn to parent by the way we were parented or by the way we observe someone we admire parenting. Unfortunately, that is the way old wives' tales and emotionally damaging parenting skills are passed from one generation to another and another and another...

What was accepted and what worked for one generation will not necessarily work and be appropriate for the current society. Today's parents have the advantage of proven advice from child development experts available in books, videos, the Internet, television, and magazines. Parent education in the form of home visitation and parenting classes is also sweeping the nation as a way of helping parents develop effective parenting skills while learning about child development. We have the results of long-term studies that help determine exactly what *effective* parenting consists of. Parents are hungry for this knowledge! We want to be good parents and raise happy, well-adjusted children if we only have the tools of knowledge and support which will help us do that.

As the parent of a new baby, you have the exciting opportunity to use this information to become the effective parent we all desire to be. A word of caution: there is no such thing as a perfect parent or a perfect child. You *will* have difficulties in your parenting. You *will* make mistakes. Your baby *will* try your patience and deprive you of sleep and personal time. Not because you are doing something wrong or because your baby is bad, but simply because he is a baby and that's what babies do. *Your Baby's Instruction Book* will help you learn what to expect and how to cope. This in turn will make life easier for both you and your baby and allow you to enjoy and treasure this very special time as your newborn enters into the family.

Since this is your new baby's "instruction book," the headings will follow the theme of other instruction manuals. Never think for a moment, however, that we consider an infant in the same light as we would a material object. A baby is a gift of God to be loved unconditionally, cared for responsibly, treasured, and respected to the fullest measure—and that is truly the purpose of this book.

<u>IMPORTANT NOTICE</u>

PREMATURITY:

If your baby was born prematurely, your pediatrician may have given you special instructions that need to be followed. Keep that in mind and make the necessary changes as you go through this book. Also adjust your baby's age to his full-term age before applying the recommendations or considering the average age range chart for milestones given in this book. For example, if your baby was born eight weeks early, adjust the expectations by two months younger. A four-month-old baby who was born eight weeks premature may be developmentally more like a two-month-old full-term infant. The difference will be less noticeable as your baby gets older. The more premature your baby, the longer you may have to make adjustments. Almost all babies are caught up by two years.

SHERRY KELLY

<u>SETTING UP</u>

Your baby will require a certain amount of clothing and equipment. You can be elaborate and spend a lot of money or be modest and spend a little money and still fill the needs of your infant. Babies outgrow things very quickly. As a result, you can find lots of almost new items at second-hand stores and garage sales. Chances are you have been "nesting" the last few months of your pregnancy and have most everything ready and waiting for your baby. There is an abundance of baby equipment on the market today. It is fun for parents to have these nice conveniences for their babies. However, don't feel you are depriving your little one if you cannot afford or do not have room for many of these extras. Many organizations will provide clothing and other items for those who need them. If you are financially troubled at this time and need assistance, call your local health department, hospital, guidance center, or cooperative extension and ask about what might be available to you. The following is a list of very basic necessities which every baby needs.

THE LAYETTE:

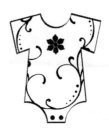

(Basic wardrobe for baby)

- 6–8 changes of clothing for day and night (a mixture of stretch suits, shirts, gowns, etc.)
- 4–6 pair of socks or booties
- 1 warm bunting with hat or hood (if during winter)
- 6–8 receiving blankets
- 2 heavy weight sleepers or sleep sacks for cool nights
- 3–4 crib sheets
- Cloth diapers or other soft cloths for burping

This along with your choice of diapers will fill the basic needs of your baby for the first couple of months. Of course, many other things, such as bibs, cute clothes for outings, sweaters, etc. are available. All clothing, whether new or used, should be washed before your baby wears them.[1] Fabric softeners and dryer sheets should not be used on infant and children's clothing because it is thought that they reduce the effectiveness of fire resistant fabrics. Most softener bottles carry a warning about this in fine print which is often overlooked.

NURSERY EQUIPMENT:

Crib.

First and foremost, keep safety in mind when shopping for nursery equipment. Your baby will spend a lot of time in his crib, and you will want to know s/he is safe. The bed should be sturdy with no loose or missing parts. The rails must be spaced no more than 2 3/8 inches apart. A quick and simple test is to see if a soda can fits between the rails. If it does, the crib is not safe.

The mattress should fit snugly with no room for baby to squeeze between it and the sides. Corner posts which extend more than one-sixteenth of an inch higher than the top edge of the crib, and decorative cutouts in the head and foot boards, should be avoided. You do not want anything that could catch your baby or his clothing. Put the crib in a safe place. Be sure any blind cords or curtain tiebacks are well out of reach and pose no danger.

Changing table.

A changing table is nice for changing your baby as well as storing clothes and supplies, but it is not a necessity. You can change baby on a bed or on a folded blanket placed on a table, dresser, or countertop. *Always* keep a hand on baby to be sure he does not fall.

Baby swing/Bouncer seat.

Although not truly a necessity, a baby swing or bouncer seat is considered a necessity by some parents. Not all babies enjoy baby swings, but those who do can be comforted in the swing during those times when mom or dad cannot conveniently hold and sooth the baby.

Never leave your baby unattended while in the swing and especially *never* leave a dog alone with a baby in a swing. The movement of the swing and the sound it makes can cause even a well-behaved family pet to injure the baby.

Highchair.

A highchair will be needed once your little one can sit well and begins to self-feed. Always buckle him in and keep a close eye on him while he is in the chair. Babies have been injured due to falling, climbing, and sliding out of highchairs.

Playpen.

If not over-used, a playpen is a benefit to busy moms and babies. It provides a safe place to put your baby for brief periods throughout the day. Do not use one that has netting wide enough for a small button to catch. If the netting gets a hole or tears, it will no longer be safe. Never leave your baby in the playpen with one side folded down as babies have been suffocated in this way.

Always follow the manufacturer's instructions for safe use of any products you buy. Be sure to fill out and return the registration card that comes with the products so the manufacturer can contact you about any recalls. Frequently look things over for any disrepair which could negate their safety. Before buying any used infant or child equipment, check with the manufacturer or the Consumer Product Safety Commission to be sure there are no problems.[2]

CAR SEAT:

One absolute necessity is an approved car seat. There are many different styles and sizes from which to pick. Look for one that appears comfortable and that has sufficient straps to keep baby secure. Also check to see how easy it will be for you to buckle and unbuckle baby as you will be putting him/her in and out of the seat often. You must have a car seat to bring your baby home from the hospital. Some organizations provide car seats for a small fee. If you would like help in locating a car seat, call your local health department or the social worker at the hospital.

The car seat must be installed properly to be effective. Many organizations such as SAFE KIDS Coalitions, Cooperative Extensions, ambulance services, and local fire departments, offer free car seat checks. Call to see what is available in your area.[3] Never use a car seat that has been in a car accident as this can weaken its effectiveness.[4]

REGISTRATION

One of the most important decisions you will make concerning your child will be the name you select. The name will affect the child his/her entire life and should be given serious consideration. A person's name can either evoke positive or negative impressions from others. Research in preparation for *The New Baby Name Survey*, a book by Bruce Lansky,[1] concluded that many names are associated with certain impressions concerning the personality of an individual. The name of any well-known person—past or present—in the news, movies, television, history, politics, etc. can cause us to unconsciously think of that person's personality and apply it to others with that name. Of course, after you get to know an individual, your original impression may be radically changed.

However, first impressions are important and can stick in the minds of those who never really get to know us. If someone hears a name before meeting the person, they will likely form an impression in response to the name alone and will treat the person accordingly at the initial encounter. For example, what images first come to your mind when you hear the names Adolph, Jezebel, Madonna, Cher, Roseanne, Oprah, Garth, or Shaq? Stay clear of names that give an immediate negative impression. You will want your child's name to have a positive or neutral influence on the way people respond.

GUIDELINES TO HELP IN CHOOSING A NAME:

1. Pick a name that you and other family members really like. Consider family names and cultural names that are connected with your heritage.

2. Think about the name carefully. Do the first, middle, and last names sound well together? Consider how the name sounds for a baby, child, teenager, young adult, and then older adult. Will it be suitable for your child throughout life?

3. Go to the library and find a book of names that gives the meanings or origins of names. Choose a name that your child will feel good about should he sometime be presented with its meaning.

4. Consider the initials of the first and last name, then the first, middle, and last name. Be sure they don't form anything that might be embarrassing.

5. A name that is clearly male or female is preferred over unisex names, which can cause confusion.

6. Avoid humorous combinations and names that are very unusual. Comments on such names can become monotonous after a while—not only for the child but for the parent also.

7. Have names selected for both a girl and a boy. Ultrasound predictions are not 100 percent accurate, and you do not want to have to come up with a name in a hurry.

BIRTH CERTIFICATE:

Before you and your baby leave the hospital, you will be asked for your baby's name as you want it recorded on the birth certificate. Be sure the spelling is accurate.

If you are a single mother, the father will not be named on the certificate unless both parents sign a paternity affidavit in front of a notary. Some hospitals offer this in the hospital, while others require you to go to the department of health a couple of weeks later. If the father is named on the birth certificate, he can be held responsible for the child financially and otherwise. He also will have equal custody rights. The child cannot be given the father's last name without the father's name listed on the certificate. However, the mother's last name can be given to the child either way. (Signing a paternity affidavit can be delayed to some time in the future and the child's last name can be changed to that of the father at that time if desired. Some states have time limits for this.)

If you were married at the time the baby was conceived, or at the time of birth, the name of the husband will be entered on the certificate as the father unless all parties sign papers that state otherwise.[2] These rules vary from state to state. If you have questions regarding the birth certificate, phone the hospital where you plan to deliver and ask to talk with the "birth certificate clerk."

Remember, some names are adorable for a little child, but your child will someday be an adult who wants to be taken seriously in his/her chosen career. Will the name you select still be appropriate? Who knows? Your child's name could someday be listed among the presidents![3]

PRESET MENU

UNIQUE INDIVIDUAL:

In some ways your baby may be exactly like one of his parents. For example, his ears may be shaped with a "crook" in them—just like his mother; or he may be "fidgety" and cannot be still—just like his father. Yet in other ways he may be as different from either of you as night is from day. Just as all people are different, your baby is one-of-a-kind. No baby ever born before or after will be the same. Every baby is born a unique individual with his own personality, likes, and dislikes. It will be your goal to get to know the baby placed in your arms and help this particular little "being" develop according to his potential. You cannot make your baby into something he is not, but by the way you respond to him, you can help him grow into a happy, functional person who is using his own personal talents to achieve and feel good about himself.[1]

SHERRY KELLY

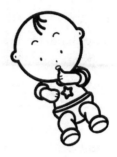

Reflexes are natural involuntary or automatic physical movements or responses. Babies are born with a number of reflexes which help in their adjustment to living outside the womb. Some of these—like gagging and blinking—will remain throughout life, but most—like the sucking and rooting reflexes—will disappear after several weeks. Others—like the stepping and grasping reflexes—will re-emerge later as consciously controlled activities.

The startle or moro reflex is often a response to a sudden noise or movement. It is characterized by the baby throwing out his arms and legs while arching his head back. He then pulls the arms and legs back in close to the body. He may cry, and he may sometimes do this in his sleep. This reflex generally fades at about eight weeks of age.

The rooting reflex is nature's way of helping the baby find food. It is characterized by baby turning toward and opening his mouth wide when his cheek is touched. If a nipple is placed in baby's mouth, his sucking reflex kicks in and allows a hungry baby to feed. The sucking reflex is present even when baby is not hungry and therefore is not always a sign of hunger. The hand-to-mouth reflex encourages babies to self-comfort by sucking their hand or fingers. The rooting, sucking, and hand-to-mouth reflexes begin to fade at around four months. Of course, by then your baby has learned to nurse for nourishment and no longer needs these primitive reflexes.

Your baby's hands are often tightly clenched as a result of the grasp reflex. As a result of this reflex, he will hold on tightly when you place your finger in his palm. This reflex fades between four and five months of age, and you will notice that baby's grasp becomes more purposeful.

The tonic neck reflex is interesting to notice. When you place your baby on his back he will turn his head to one side and his arm on that side will straighten out. The opposite arm will be bent as in a fencing position. There is no obvious purpose to this reflex, and it disappears between five and seven months of age.[2]

SYSTEM DIAGRAM

APGAR SCORES:

Your baby's heart rate, breathing, muscle tone, reflex response, and color will be checked and given a score at one minute after birth and again at five minutes after birth. This Apgar score gives the doctor an immediate indication of your baby's general condition and alerts him/her to any special needs your baby may have. Most infants score between 8 and 10 with 10 being the perfect score. (This testing system gets its name from its creator, Virginia Apgar.)[1]

SHERRY KELLY

NORMAL CHARACTERISTICS OF NEWBORNS:

1. Infants are born with two soft spots, or fontanels, on their heads. These will close up between the ages of three to twelve months, as the baby grows.[2]

2. Because babies' heads are rather soft and pliable to allow them to pass more easily through the birth canal, they may appear misshapen or bruised for a few days. Depending on the birth process, it could take several months for their heads to round out.

3. Your baby's sense of smell and hearing are well-developed at birth. Studies show that newborns can actually distinguish between their own mother's breast milk and another's by scent.[3] Babies also become familiar with their mother's voice while in the womb and are naturally calmed by it after birth.[4] On the

other hand, your baby's sight will be limited and blurred for a while. He can focus best at a distance of eight to fifteen inches.[5] Babies are naturally attracted to people, and they will look longer at the human face than anything else.

4. The newborn's bowel movements the first few days are made up of a thick, dark, substance referred to as meconium. Once the meconium is eliminated, the movements will become softer and turn yellowish in color.[6]

5. Your baby will express his needs by crying. You can help your baby feel loved and secure by filling his needs accurately and as quickly as possible. Don't worry about "spoiling." Today, it is recommended that parents cater to their baby's every whim for the first three or four months. This will lay the foundation for a happy, secure, and less demanding older baby.[7]

JAUNDICE

Babies are born with more red blood cells than they need, and as the body breaks these down, a chemical known as bilirubin builds up. Because baby's liver is immature, it has a hard time filtering this bilirubin efficiently. As a result, many normal, healthy infants will develop a yellowish tinge to their skin and the whites of the eyes for the first few days. Your doctor may recommend placing your baby under special lights as treatment. Her eyes will be covered to protect them from the brightness. If your baby is listless or becomes very yellow, or if the jaundice persists, check with your doctor.[8]

SPECIAL NEWBORN DANGERS:

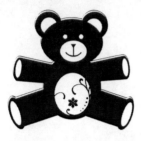

Don't underestimate your baby's abilities. Even a newborn infant may wiggle and squirm from one place to another. Never leave a baby unattended on a bed or sofa. Many caregivers have felt safe in doing so only to experience the fear and guilt of having the baby fall to the floor. Babies can also become wedged between the sofa cushions or pillows and smother. In recent years, waterbeds have been discovered to be extremely hazardous to infants. The baby can become trapped between the water-filled mattress and frame and suffocate.

Always place your baby safely in his crib or playpen to sleep. Keep his crib free of pillows, stuffed animals, and heavy blankets. Babies have been known to squirm underneath or against these and are unable to breathe. Never leave your baby on a soft or fluffy surface like a pillow, sheepskin, or beanbag [9]

Until your baby can roll over freely, it is recommended that you always place him on his back to sleep. In the 1980s a team of researchers discovered that other countries where babies routinely slept on their backs had fewer incidents of Sudden Infant Death Syndrome (SIDS). The American Academy of Pediatrics began recommending that babies sleep on their backs in 1992. The results were astounding. By 1998 the SIDS rate in the United States had dropped by forty percent. As more parents complied to this new recommendation, the rate continued to decline. By 2005 there were more than fifty percent fewer deaths diagnosed as SIDS.[10]

It is important to place your baby on his stomach during the day when he is awake and you are present to keep an eye on him. This will help to strengthen his arm and shoulder muscles as well as helping to keep his head well rounded.

SOME ASSEMBLY
MAY BE REQUIRED

CIRCUMCISION:

If your baby is a boy, you will need to decide whether or not to have him circumcised. At birth the penis has skin which covers, or almost covers, the tip of the penis. Circumcision is a minor surgical procedure which removes this skin.

In recent years there have been a lot of differing opinions about the need for circumcision. There is compelling evidence which suggests that uncircumcised males are more likely to develop urinary tract infections, have a greater risk for contracting sexually transmitted diseases and HIV, and are susceptible to the rare condition of cancer of the penis. There is also inconclusive evidence which indicates that cervical cancer may be more common among females whose partners are uncircumcised.[1]

Aside from medical issues, circumcision may be done for religious reasons or simply as a matter of family tradition or preference. Some parents believe that circumcision is unnecessary and choose not to subject their infant to this surgery which the American Academy of Pediatrics considers to be elective.[2]

Discuss the pros and cons of circumcision with your doctor to be certain you have all the latest information before making your decision. There is little risk involved when circumcision is performed on healthy infants. However, if your baby has any illness at birth, is premature, or has any congenital birth defects or blood problems, the probability for complications increases and should be considered.

In years past, circumcision was often done without anesthesia, but today most doctors routinely use a local anesthesia to minimize the baby's discomfort. Ask your doctor about this ahead of time just to be sure.

INSTALLATION

EARLY BONDING AND ADAPTING:

Bonding is often used to refer to the contact time immediately following birth when parents and babies begin their attachment. While the first minutes spent with your newborn are truly special, "bonding" or developing a feeling of belonging is actually a gradual, long-term process. Some mothers experience a rush of love for their infant at birth while others need more time to feel this closeness. The feeling of attachment comes as they hold, talk, feed, and care for their baby and watch him respond.

At best, the first few weeks with a new baby are both exhilarating and exhausting. The first days are filled with the excitement of sharing your good news with friends and relatives. After several days of visitors, phone calls, and little rest, you may be so tired you wonder how you can survive another day. Reality begins to set in, and you realize you have become a parent!

SHERRY KELLY

Keep things at home as simple as possible. Mom's body needs time to recover from pregnancy and childbirth. The baby needs all the time and energy you can muster. New parents often feel overwhelmed with the needs of a newborn. Feeding, changing, and calming this new little being is a constant around-the-clock occurrence. You will soon discover that parenting is full of ups and downs. At times you will feel so much love and pride in your baby, you think you cannot contain it, while at other times, you may be extremely tired, stressed, and frustrated by your baby's crying.

ADJUSTMENT:

As you and your baby get to know each other, you will begin to settle into a routine. It will be quite apparent that baby has made his place in the home. His "things" are spread all over the house, and life now centers around his needs. He has changed your role and the roles of all others in your household. The atmosphere in the home will affect your baby's behavior. A calm home leads to a calmer baby, where as a chaotic home leads to a fussier baby. It is to everyone's advantage to adjust as smoothly as possible into your new roles and routines. (A baby will pick up any tension and act accordingly.) Babies are very sensitive to the way they are handled and the tone of voice people use with them and each other. To feel secure a baby must be gently held, talked to, and touched. His needs should be met quickly and completely.

When baby is about three months old, things will have eased up a bit. He is waiting a little longer between feedings and sleeping a little longer at a time. He may even be sleeping through the night. Mom's body is also beginning to get back to normal, and both parents should be feeling a little less tired. However, the luxury of free time and uninterrupted meals, work, and television programs are a thing of the past and the not-so-near future. Life has also taken on new meaning for you. Your precious little child depends on you for his every need, and his smile is worth more to you than anything money could buy.[1]

<u>POWER ON</u>

HOW BABY LEARNS TO TRUST:

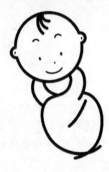

Your baby's every need was filled continuously while in the womb. He didn't know hot or cold. He did not experience hunger. Although it is thought he could hear muffled sounds and even distinguish light through the mother's uterus, he was protected from bright lights and noise. At birth he is forced to make a transition from the ideal environment of the uterus to the confusion of the outside world. What a traumatic experience that must be! Soon baby is placed against his mother's warm skin and covered with a blanket. He blinks his eyes until they become somewhat accustomed to light. He looks into his parents' faces and hears their voices, with which he is familiar. Just about the time he thinks maybe things are okay, he is whisked away to be weighed, measured, and have drops placed in his eyes. He soon falls asleep exhausted, and when he awakes he feels his first pangs of hunger. He does not like what he feels. He does what nature has equipped him to do—he

---

cries! If someone comes quickly to fill his need, he will be reassured once again and know he will be taken care of. If he is left to cry, he may become frustrated, frightened, insecure, and angry.

Dr. Karp, in his book titled, *The Happiest Baby on the Block*, wisely explains his method of trying to recreate an environment for your newborn that is similar to the womb your baby was so comfortable in. To do this he recommends his "5 S's."[1]

1. *Swaddling* (wrapping your baby snuggly in a light blanket) to provide the continuous touching and support she felt in her Momma's womb.

2. Placing your infant on her *Side* or *Stomach* (only while you are holding her, always return her to her back when placing her into her crib).

3. *Shushing Sounds* or sounds that mimic what your baby heard while inside the womb. This can be as simple as a soft verbal "shhh" or using some sort of "white noise" such as a fan or recorded "womb sounds."

4. *Swinging*: Provide the continual motion your baby felt while in the womb.

5. *Sucking*, notes Dr. Karp, "triggers the calming reflex and releases natural chemicals within the brain." This can be provided with the breast, bottle, pacifier, or finger.

Dr. Karp's method will help all babies adjust to life outside the womb.

Years ago parents were told that if they picked up their babies every time they cried they would become spoiled or demanding. Mothers were instructed to let their babies cry or they would soon expect mom to drop everything and come running every time they whimpered. Today, child development experts believe just the opposite to be true.

In 1972 Ainsworth, Bell, and Stayton studied two groups of babies.[2] One group's mothers met their needs quickly and gave them lots of attention. The other group was allowed to cry until it was convenient for mom to attend to them. The babies were followed through toddlerhood and the results were clear. The babies whose mothers were quick to respond felt secure, cried very little, and were patient to wait for mom's attention. It seems these babies were assured from the beginning that their needs would be met and they would be taken care of. As a result these babies had developed "basic trust"—a feeling of security which is an essential human need.

From the newborn's point of view, life becomes either good or bad in relation to the way his basic needs are supplied. He tries to communicate these needs by crying. It is up to the caregiver to respond appropriately. Is baby hungry? Does he just need to suck? Is he sleepy or lonely or bored? Could he be too hot or too cold? Is a wet diaper making him uncomfortable?

Does he need a quiet place to relax? When his needs are consistently met and he is held, cuddled, and talked to, he begins to feel loved and valued.

Any baby nurse can tell you that differences are immediately noticed among the newborns in the hospital nursery. Some babies are quiet, sleep a lot, and have to be awakened for feedings. Other babies are wiggly, awake often, and require more attention. Some babies snuggle up next to the body when they are picked up, while others tend to stiffen up and prefer to be held out away from the body. Becoming sensitive to your baby's temperament will help you respond in an appropriate way. For example, holding a non-cuddler baby close might only frustrate him and cause him to cry harder.

Ideas:

Ask other moms what their babies are like. Ask about their sleep patterns and whether they like to be cuddled. What things do the babies particularly like and dislike? Ask your mom what you were like as an infant. Ask the mother of your baby's father what he was like as an infant. Notice the temperaments of babies you come in contact with and try to think about how each would respond to different situations.[3]

MAINTENANCE

BREASTFEEDING:

Health care professionals agree that breastfeeding is the best possible start you can give your baby. All new mothers are encouraged to breastfeed their babies. Two days are better than none at all. One month is still better, etc. Following are some of the advantages of breastfeeding.

1. A human mother's milk is the perfect natural food for a human baby. It contains superior nutrition in the right proportions. It is all that baby needs for the first four to six months.

2. During the first couple of days after birth, the breasts produce colostrum, which is unique to the baby's early needs. It is rich, high in protein, and low in sugar and fat. It is easy to digest and full of antibodies to protect against a wide variety of diseases. It also helps "clean baby out."

3. Breast milk enhances cognitive development in the infant (higher intelligence).[1]

4. Babies who are breastfed have less diaper rash, fewer colds, and some protection from allergies.[2]

5. Breastfeeding is convenient. There are no bottles to wash or formulas to prepare. It is always ready to feed at the right temperature.

6. Comparing the price of the extra calories consumed by a nursing mother to the high cost of formula, breast milk is much cheaper.

7. Breastfeeding helps the mother's uterus and hormonal elevations get back to normal.

8. Breastfeeding can be a pleasurable experience for a mother and her baby promoting emotional benefits such as mother-infant closeness and calmness.

9. Mothers who breastfeed have a reduced incidence of breast cancer and osteoporosis.[3]

Almost all mothers can breastfeed. The size of the breast does not matter. Small- or large-breasted mothers alike produce as much milk as their babies require. Women with flat or inverted nipples can also be successful at breastfeeding. Avoid using soap or cream on your breasts as these destroy the natural lubricant excreted by the breast's glands. This natural lubricant protects the nipples during pregnancy and breastfeeding.

Although breastfeeding is natural, it is not something you and your baby will automatically know how to do. You will both be a little awkward at first. Ideally the infant is put to breast immediately after birth. Today, many hospitals have lactation educators who instruct new mothers, get them off to a good start, and answer any questions.

Steps to Start Breastfeeding:[4]

1. Baby should be awake, and mother should be as comfortable as possible—in either a lying or sitting position.

2. Gently hold your breast in one hand while baby is positioned facing you (tummy to tummy).

3. Touch baby's cheek or lips with your nipple until he opens his mouth *wide*.

4. When he opens wide, quickly place your breast inside his mouth, putting the nipple over baby's tongue and pulling baby closer at the same time.

5. Check to be sure that baby has the whole nipple plus at least one inch of the dark area around it in his mouth. *This is very important for successful breastfeeding*. If baby does not have enough of the breast in his mouth, slip your little finger into the corner of his mouth to break the suction and then try again. If you can hear baby swallowing, he is nursing properly.

A new baby needs to be fed every two to four hours around the clock. Respond to early signs of hunger such as rooting or sucking on hands, and do not wait until the baby is crying. It is more difficult for a new baby to begin breastfeeding when he is crying. Breastfeed your baby at both breasts every feeding for at least five to ten minutes each. Alternate the breast with which you begin. Some mothers find it convenient to slip a loose rubber band or bracelet over the wrist of the side to begin with, as a reminder. You can try burping your baby after each breast by holding him upright and gently patting or rubbing his back. If after several minutes he does not burp, he probably does not need to and can be put to the other breast.

During the first few weeks, your baby should be fed eight to ten times every twenty-four hours.[5] *The amount of milk you produce depends on the amount of sucking your baby does. The more baby sucks, the more milk you will have available at the next feeding.* If your baby has about six to eight wet diapers and at least two bowel movements each day, he is getting enough breast milk. As the newborn grows, the normal frequency of the bowel movements will change and will vary widely from one baby to another. After about four to six weeks, some breast-fed babies will have only one stool every three or four days or more and still be considered normal.

If your baby was born prematurely, you may be unable to feed him/her directly for awhile. It will be important for you to pump regularly to build up and maintain your milk supply. Your breast milk is ideally suited for your baby and will help him/her grow and mature in the best possible way. Ask the lactation nurse to suggest a good breast pump and guide you through this process.

In general babies need no feedings other than the breast while in the hospital. A bottle nipple may confuse a baby who is just learning to breastfeed. In a few weeks, if baby is breastfeeding well, you can begin giving him a pacifier and expressed milk from a bottle on occasion.

Three to five days after birth, your milk supply increases and your breasts will become hard and full. This is referred to as engorgement or "your milk coming in." Although engorgement is a positive sign, it can be rather uncomfortable. Engorgement is a *temporary* condition lasting only a day or two. During engorgement, breastfeed at least every two hours for ten minutes at each breast. Between feedings cool wet cloths or ice packs applied around your breasts may make you more comfortable. Just before feeding, place warm wet wash cloths on your breasts and express a few drops of milk with your fingers to soften the nipple area and make it easier for baby to latch on.

In a couple of weeks, breastfeeding will become much easier and more comfortable. Then just about the time you think everything is going well, you may notice baby acting as though he is still hungry after feeding. Do not jump to the conclusion that your milk is drying up as this is generally a sign your baby is going through a growth-spurt and just needs a little more milk. Your milk supply will soon increase to fill his needs.

La Leche League is an organization that provides information and encouragement to breastfeeding mothers and mothers-to-be. Ask around to find a group that meets in your area.[6]

Breastfeeding takes a little extra work in the beginning, but mothers who stick it out find it well worth the effort. Breastfeeding is a special gift only you can give your baby![7]

BOTTLE-FEEDING:

Not all mothers choose to breastfeed. You may have adopted or you may have medical reasons or other causes that prevent it. For whatever reason, if you have made this choice, you can be reassured that feeding your baby formula is a healthy alternative.

Ask your pediatrician to guide you in your choice of baby formulas. Most infant formulas are available in ready-to-feed bottles but they are more expensive than liquid concentrates or powder. Follow carefully the instructions on the container for mixing. This is very important to be sure your baby gets all the nutrients he needs.

There is some question about the safety of plastic bottles which contain the manmade chemical, Bisphenol A (BPA). To be on the safe side, it is recommended that you choose bottles which are BPA free.[8],[9]

You can sterilize bottles and nipples by placing them in boiling water for five to ten minutes. This

---

may not be necessary if you use a dishwasher. Ask your pediatrician's advice about the need for sterilization, as the view on this has changed over the years and may depend on your local water supply. Your pediatrician may recommend boiling the water you add to the concentrated or powdered formula.

Formula can be fed to your baby either cool or at room temperature; however, if you want to duplicate the temperature of breast milk, you will need to warm the bottle. The simplest way is just to set it in a cup of hot tap water for a few minutes. Warming the bottle in the microwave is thought to cause a breakdown in nutrients and therefore should not be done. Always check the temperature of a warmed bottle by shaking a drop or two on the inside of your forearm. If it is too hot, let it cool and then check it again.

Newborn babies have tiny tummies and can only hold two to three ounces of formula at a feeding. Your baby will need to be fed every three to four hours. As he grows, gradually increase the amount of formula given at each feeding. By six months of age, your baby will be drinking about six to eight ounces of formula at each feeding with about four or five feedings in a twenty-four-hour day.[10]

Hold your baby slightly upright during feedings, being careful to keep the nipple full of milk. This will help prevent air from entering your baby's sensitive system and causing painful gas. Keep a cloth diaper or something similar handy during feedings to catch dribbles. Do *not* prop the bottle to feed as this can cause gas and choking, and also denies your baby the nurturing needed for healthy development. *Never* put your baby to bed with a bottle even when he can hold it himself. The formula may pool around his teeth and cause decay. This condition is known as nursing-bottle syndrome and can be very painful as well as expensive to treat and to correct. Drinking while lying down also can contribute to recurring ear infections.[11]

To avoid future weaning difficulties, do not let your baby carry his bottle around as he gets bigger. Let him drink from it when he needs nourishment and then put the bottle away until the next feeding.

Do not feed infants under the age of twelve months regular milk. Even though most baby formulas are cow's milk based, they are dramatically different than regular cow's milk we buy at the store for children and adults to drink. Cow's milk contains high concentrations of protein and minerals, which can put a strain on a baby's kidneys and cause dehydration. It also does not contain enough iron and vitamin C and could lead to iron-deficiency anemia in some babies. Do not change your baby's formula before discussing it with your doctor.[12]

Babies generally get all the water they need from breast milk or formula. Drinking too much water is dangerous for infants.

BURPING:

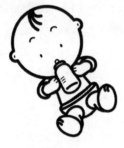

For breast-fed babies, burp after each breast, and for bottle-fed babies, burp after every two or three ounces. Burp your baby more often if he begins to fuss or squirm. You can hold him over your shoulder and gently pat his back or sit him on your lap supporting his head and chest with one hand while patting or rubbing his back with the other. Protect your clothing from possible spit up with a cloth diaper or burp cloths.

SPITTING UP:

Spitting up is a common occurrence for babies. Their little digestive systems are new and sensitive. It usually happens shortly after feedings and is generally nothing to be concerned about. Avoid jostling the baby too soon after he eats. As baby grows, he should spit up less and less often. Use a cloth diaper or other absorbent cloth to catch the mess, especially while burping. If, however, your baby is spitting up large amounts, talk to your pediatrician.

THE UMBILICAL CORD:

The umbilical cord was your baby's lifeline while in the womb. Once baby is born and breathing on her own, the cord is no longer needed. It is painlessly clamped and cut at birth. The clamp will be removed within twenty-four to forty-eight hours, and the cord will then continue to dry up and shrink until it drops off in about ten days to three weeks. Keep your baby's diaper folded down below the umbilical cord. This will help keep it dry and clean. Use a cotton swab dipped in rubbing alcohol to gently wash around the base of the cord. Keep an eye on the area, and if you notice any pus, oozing, or red skin at the base of the cord, call your doctor as it could be a sign of infection.[13]

SHERRY KELLY

Give your baby only sponge baths until the cord falls off. Have everything you need ready before getting your baby for the bath. Place him on a folded towel or blanket in a warm area. Use warm water in a sink or bowl, and use a cloth to wash baby beginning with his face and hair. Use only a water-dampened cloth for his face and use a small amount of baby shampoo to gently massage his scalp and hair. Rinse the hair well by holding his head over the basin and gently and carefully pouring water over the hair. For baby's comfort, keep him wrapped up and only expose the area you are washing (this may be difficult because of baby's movement). Continue washing using a gentle baby soap until the bath is complete. Pay special attention to all the creases and make sure they are well washed, rinsed, and dried. If your baby cries during the bath, just stay calm and talk soothingly while you go through the process.

After the cord falls off, you can place your baby

directly into about two inches of water in a baby tub or sink. Check the water temperature with your wrist before putting your baby in. Always keep a hand on your infant during baths and *never* leave him unattended, not even for a second. If you need to leave the area for any reason, wrap the towel around your baby and take her with you. Babies only need to be bathed two or three times a week during the first year.[14] Do not use powders or lotions during the first month. Thereafter, baby lotions and powders should be used sparingly. If using powder, use caution to prevent baby from breathing the powder dust.

CRADLE CAP:

Cradle cap is a scaly rash that often develops on a new baby's scalp. You can help keep it to a minimum by shampooing his hair frequently using a mild baby shampoo. Even if your baby has only a bit of fine hair, use a soft baby brush daily. Cradle cap generally clears up after a few months, but if the rash gets worse or spreads to the face, neck, or crease areas, contact your doctor.

DIAPER RASH:

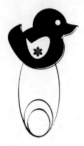

To prevent diaper rash, change your baby often. Wash the diaper area with a cloth and warm water after each bowel movement. Baby wipes can be used after the first month. If a rash does develop, apply petroleum jelly or ointment to make baby more comfortable as he heals. If it does not clear up in a couple of days, consult your pediatrician.

Babies' faces get chapped easily, especially in the winter due to the cold, dry weather. Excessive drooling also causes the mouth area and chin to get red and raw. If your baby has a runny nose, it too can become raw and uncomfortable. All of these can be soothed by applying petroleum jelly to the affected areas before putting your baby to bed. Lotions sometime sting when applied to raw skin and may irritate the area further.

NAIL CARE:

Newborns have little control over their hands and may accidentally scratch their faces. Their nails grow quickly in the first few weeks, and you may need to trim them as often as twice a week. Most parents find the easiest way to accomplish this is to use a nail clipper while their baby is asleep. Use extreme caution with the clippers so as not to cut the tip of baby's delicate fingers.

HICCUPS:

No one seems to know just why babies hiccup so often, beginning even in the womb. Some say it is because they are over-stimulated or stressed and need to be soothed in a quiet area. An old wives tale states that it is simply a sign they are growing. Whatever the reason, even though they get the hiccups fairly frequently, they don't usually last more than a few minutes at a time. As the baby grows, they become less frequent.[15]

PACIFIERS:

Pacifiers can soothe your baby between feedings when he just needs to suck. If you are nursing, wait until breast feeding is well established to introduce a pacifier, so you do not risk confusing your baby. Choose a small pacifier which is dishwasher safe. Buy several so you will always have a clean one when needed. Always keep safety in mind. Do not tie the pacifier around your baby's neck. Check each pacifier often to be sure it is sturdy and discard any which have gotten soft or have broken. Do not use regular baby bottle nipples for a pacifier as babies have been known to suck them into their throats and choke.

SHERRY KELLY

WHEN TO START ON CEREAL, JUICE, AND BABY FOOD:

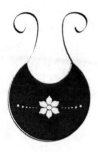

Babies are born with a *tongue-thrust* reflex which causes them to push against a spoon or anything placed in the mouth including food. They begin to lose this reflex at about four months of age. That is one of the reasons that four months is the recommended age to begin babies on iron-fortified rice cereal. Another reason is because at about this age their salivary glands are beginning to produce more saliva.

Use a small spoon to feed your baby solid food and be especially patient as she learns this new way of eating. Some parents try putting the cereal in a bottle to feed, but this can drastically increase the amount of food she takes in and lead to excessive weight gain. Furthermore, it is important for baby to get used to the process of eating using the mouth, tongue, chewing, and swallowing. Placing a bib on baby before feeding will make cleanup easier. Make mealtime a pleasant time and offer very small amounts—just a spoon full or two—to begin. If she cries and turns away when you try to feed her, don't force the issue. Wait a while and try again.

Vegetables and fruits can be given to baby at about six months; meats and mashed table foods at about eight months; and egg yolk and finger foods at about ten months. Wait at least three days between new foods to watch for any adverse reactions.

Two to three ounces of juice can be introduced—along with drinking from a sippy cup—at about six months. The American Academy of Pediatrics recommends giving your baby a limited amount of juice once a day. Offer the juice in a training cup. Read the label and be sure you are getting juice with no sugar or artificial coloring additives. Keep in mind that even one hundred percent juice is very sweet. Too much juice may lead to babies not eating the foods they need, becoming overweight, having diarrhea,[16] and developing cavities.[17]

It is always a temptation to give your baby little tastes of coke or tea, etc. while you are drinking. This is not in your baby's best interest. It is not good for him, so do not start it.

Do not feed babies under one year of age egg whites, honey, or peanut butter. If you give egg whites or peanut butter too early, your baby could develop allergies, and honey can cause infant botulism.[18]

Until your baby is four years old, any round, firm, foods are considered choking hazards and should not be given unless they are chopped completely. These include hot dogs, raw vegetables, and chunks of fruit. Moreover, some common favorites are some of the most dangerous and should not be given to any child under the age of four years. The following snacks put babies and children under four years old at a high risk for choking: [19]

- Nuts and seeds
- Whole grapes
- Hard, gooey, or sticky candy
- Popcorn
- Chunks of peanut butter
- Chewing gum

Insist that toddlers and children eat only while sitting in a highchair or at the table. Walking, lying down, or playing around while eating also leads to choking.

WEANING:

Weaning should be a gradual process beginning at around eight or nine months. If you have been giving your baby his juice in a training cup, he will be fairly comfortable drinking from a cup by this age. Begin by substituting formula in his cup for one midday bottle feeding and tell him what a big boy he is to drink from his cup like mommy and daddy.

After you decide to replace a bottle with a cup, do not give in to his fussing for a bottle. It will be easier in the long run if you stand firm and encourage drinking from the cup. Give him a few days to adjust to one feeding without a bottle and then eliminate an additional daytime bottle, and then another until he is down to one bottle at bedtime at around twelve months. This final step in the weaning process will be much easier if you have never put your baby to bed with a bottle. Substitute a cup for the bedtime feeding. Let your baby help give away or pack away all the bottles and nipples. If baby knows there are no more bottles available, he will adjust more quickly.

Weaning is seldom easy, and many parents want to put it off until their baby is older. However, if you wait much past the first birthday, baby becomes so dependent on nursing from the breast or bottle that it seems to be even more difficult the longer you wait.

Once your baby is a year old, you can switch to regular whole milk. You may want to mix it half and half with formula for a few days so your baby can get used to the taste in a subtle way. Your baby should have whole milk until age two, and then you can ask your doctor about switching him to two percent milk.

NOISE REDUCTION

CRYING:

Crying is the primary way a baby communicates his needs. He may be saying he is hungry, cold, over-stimulated, tired, bored, hurting, needing a diaper change, or simply needing to be held. It is up to the parent to figure out what the baby's present need is and then to fill it as quickly as possible. Remember that your baby's every need was cared for constantly while in the womb. He was continually being held, kept clean and warm, and fed—and all in a dimly lit protected environment. When he cries, all of these things should be considered. (See Dr. Karp's 5 S's listed in the Power On section.)

Baby's first three to four months are a time of transition. Always react calmly and handle your baby gently when he is crying as this will help to soothe him. The more we nurture and soothe him during this time, the better adjusted he will be later

COLIC:

Colic is unexplained crying which occurs frequently and for extended periods. It is intense crying that is hard to soothe and usually happens in the evening when everyone is tired. It is sometimes difficult to tell the difference between colic and sickness. If your baby has any signs of sickness, be sure to contact the doctor. Babies with colic are otherwise healthy babies who cry for extended periods with no obvious reason. They often are tense and have clenched fists with their legs curled up as if they are in pain.

It is hard to see your baby in distress and not know how to help. Therefore, the continual crying that accompanies the colic can be very frustrating and upsetting for the whole family. Remind yourself that your baby's crying is not your or your baby's fault and that you are doing all you can. Try to remain as calm and relaxed as possible as this will help to calm your baby. When you feel yourself getting stressed, hand your baby over to another adult for a while or, if this is not possible, gently wrap your baby in a blanket and place him in his bed for a little while. Remind yourself that colic does not last forever, and by the time your baby is three to four months old, most of this type of crying will end.

SLEEP, STATES OF CONSCIOUSNESS, AND CUES:[1]

While crying is the most obvious way a newborn communicates, there are other ways that are much more subtle. The infant has six states of consciousness and gives us cues which not all parents are aware of. Once you understand these six states, you will be more sensitive to your baby's signals and give your infant the needed responses to each.

1. **Quiet Alert.** When your baby is quiet alert, his eyes are wide open, he is still and looks directly into your face. Your baby is saying, "Talk to me, I am listening."

2. **Active Alert.** When your baby is active alert, he is moving, looking about, and making small sounds. He is interested in things around him but pays little attention to your face. Your baby may be about to get hungry

or fussy. (If you are in a store, it might be time to prepare to leave.)

3. **Crying.** Crying is the next state and one that can sometimes be avoided if you respond appropriately to the previous states.

4. **Drowsiness.** Drowsiness occurs both when your baby is waking up and when he is falling asleep. He may continue to move, smile, or frown. His eyelids are droopy and his eyes have a dull, glazed appearance. This is a good state for your baby to be in when you put him to bed. It is important that babies learn to fall asleep in their cribs. If baby is always sound asleep when placed in the crib, he will cry for help in getting back to sleep when he wakes up. If the last thing baby sees before falling asleep is his crib, he will more likely go back to sleep on his own when he wakes up during the night.

5. **Quiet sleep.** Newborns sleep about sixteen to eighteen hours of the day and night. About half of this time is spent in quiet sleep. The baby is at full rest, there are no movements other than a rare startle, and his breathing is very regular. Baby is sleeping soundly and if moved from place to place, may remain asleep.

6. **Active sleep.** The other half of his sleep time is in active sleep or restless sleep. In this state there is occasional body activity, breathing is

irregular, and the eyes will often move under the lids (REM). It is unknown if babies dream during this state the way adults do. Baby may make faces or chewing and sucking movements. Baby may wake up if moved during this time.

OPERATING PRECAUTIONS

BABY BLUES:

As many as 50 to 70 percent of new mothers experience some form of baby blues, which is a mild form of depression characterized by the new mom's crying easily, being irritable, and feeling sad. The cause is most likely a combination of things like the mother's hormones being out of balance, lack of sleep, and the stress that comes along with having a new baby in the family. The baby blues may come and go anytime during the baby's first year. The new mother needs a little extra understanding, rest, and support during this time, and the blues usually pass in a few days. Prolonged depression may be more serious, and your doctor should be consulted.[1]

Although not often noted, new dads sometimes experience a form of depression also. Dads sometimes feel neglected, have concerns about their increased responsibilities, and suffer the same stress and lack of

SHERRY KELLY

sleep that new moms do. Both parents may have some unfounded guilt and shame for their feelings which makes things worse.

SAFETY PRECAUTIONS

Webster defines "safety" as "the state of being safe." [1]
There are many things we can do as
parents to be sure our child remains safe.

SAFE SLEEP:

To keep your baby safe during sleep, always place him in a safe crib which meets all current safety standards. Railings should be no farther apart than 2 3/8 inches. If a soda can fits between the rails, there is too much space. There should be no corner posts which extend more than 1/16 of an inch higher than the top edge of the crib.[2] Many older cribs are unsafe and should not be used.

The mattress should be firm and fit tightly against the sides. The sheet should also fit tightly. Do not have any pillows or toys in the crib with baby. Do not hang blankets, coats, etc. over the sides of the crib as these could fall into the bed with your baby. Use only a light blanket to cover baby up. Be certain no one smokes in your home or around the baby. Always place your baby on his back to sleep. Put the crib in a safe place and away from window curtain ties or shade cords.

Beware of the danger of falling asleep with your baby. Many infants have suffocated while sleeping with a family member.

GENERAL SAFETY RULES FOR KEEPING YOUR BABY SAFE:

- Always place your baby in a safety-approved car seat for travel. Be sure it is installed according to the directions and that your baby is buckled in exactly as instructed. Be aware that a seat used during an accident may no longer be safe and should be discarded.

- Protect your baby from extreme temperatures. Especially keep your baby out of direct sun light and after six months use sunscreen when you will have him out of doors.

- Keep plastic bags, balloons, and all soft plastics well away from your baby.

- Never leave your baby alone in the house.

- Never leave your baby alone in a car. Leaving a baby or child in a car puts them at a high

---

SHERRY KELLY

risk of being kidnapped or dying from heat. Just do not do it - ever.

- Never leave your baby's sight when he is in the bathtub.

- Never leave your infant unattended on a sofa, adult bed, or on a dressing table, etc.

- Never leave family pets unattended around your baby.

- Do not place ribbons, necklaces, etc. around the baby's neck.

- Do not put anything in your baby's hair that she could choke on.

- Keep all small objects away from baby. Anything that can fit through a toilet paper roll is too small to be safe.

- Be sure your home has working smoke detectors.

- Upstairs windows must have locks or guards to protect from falls.

- Select only experienced babysitters and licensed childcare facilities.

- When you have your baby with you at the store, be sure he is strapped in if you put him in the seat of the shopping cart. Never turn your back on him while he is in the cart and be sure he remains seated at all times. Many little ones have been injured when they fell from a cart or had a cart tip over while they were inside.

NEVER SHAKE A BABY:

Shaking a baby or child can lead to brain damage or death. Do not use shaking to burp your baby. Do not allow people to toss baby in the air while playing. Never shake your baby out of anger. Be sure all family members and caregivers are aware of the dangers of shaking.[3]

BABY PROOFING YOUR HOME:

When your baby begins to spend time on the floor and to scoot and crawl, you will need to baby proof your home. This means there is nothing within his reach that is a danger to him. Get down on baby's level and check every nook and cranny for any small objects that could be choking hazards, anything sharp, anything that could get hot, and anything electrical. Look for cords or anything that could be pulled down or pulled over onto baby.

Are all medications and plants well out of reach? Are all cleaning products placed on high shelves or locked up? Are all wastebaskets out of baby's reach? Is there anything around which contains water, including animal dishes, mop buckets, or ice chests? Be aware that many babies have also drowned in toilets. Use secure gates to protect your baby from steps and unsafe areas. Attach out-of-reach locks on all exterior doors and other places where needed.

SHERRY KELLY

Check your home frequently as your baby becomes more mobile. Safety needs will change as your baby grows. Check all furniture to be sure it does not tip easily if baby should try to pull up to it or climb it. Television sets have been pulled over on top of many curious and busy toddlers.

The hinged lids of toy chests, ice chests, laundry hampers, etc., have been known to fall on the necks of babies just learning to pull up. The baby may then lose his footing and strangle. Special care should be taken to keep these away from your baby. Also check your baby's toys regularly to be sure they are not broken or unsafe.[4]

If you live in a house or apartment built before 1978, you may have lead-based paint. Lead can get into your baby's system and damage his health. Be sure your baby does not chew on windowsills, etc., and wash your baby's hands frequently. Look for peeling or chipping paint and keep it cleaned up. If you suspect a problem, you can have your baby tested for blood lead levels (BLL). Old furniture and pottery may also contain lead and should not be around your baby. Be careful about choosing your baby's toys because some older toys and even new ones that were made overseas contain lead.[5]

TROUBLE SHOOTING

IMMUNIZATIONS AND WELL-BABY CHECKUPS:

To keep your baby healthy, follow your pediatrician's recommendation for well-baby checkups and immunizations. This should go to the top of your priority list. Required immunizations change from time to time depending on diseases being eradicated and new vaccines being developed. Be sure you have the latest information on this.

Talk with your pediatrician about any concerns you may have. Your well-baby checkup is also a great time to ask your doctor questions about what your baby should be eating, her development, sleeping patterns, etc.

HOW TO TAKE YOUR BABY'S TEMPERATURE:[1]

- Use a rectal thermometer.

- Shake the mercury down below the ninety-six degrees (thirty-five degrees centigrade) mark.

- Clean the bulb end with alcohol or soap and water and rinse with cool water.

- Apply a small amount of petroleum jelly to the bulb end.

- Place your baby tummy down on your lap or any firm surface. Keep one hand firmly on baby's back and hold him as still as possible.

- Insert the lubricated bulb end of the thermometer a half inch to one inch into the anal opening. Hold the thermometer firmly. Keep your fingers close to baby's bottom so that when he pushes, the thermometer cannot go any deeper into your baby.

- Hold it in place for two minutes before removing it to read.

- A rectal reading over 100.4 degrees Fahrenheit (38 degrees Celsius) may indicate fever.

WHEN TO CALL THE DOCTOR:

If you notice any change in your baby's appetite, skin color, bowel movements, breathing, or if your baby becomes lethargic, vomits, or runs a fever, you should contact your doctor. When it comes to a young baby's health, do not take chances. If you think your baby may be sick, call your doctor.

<u>LIMITED WARRANTY</u>

GROWTH AND DEVELOPMENT:

You will see dramatic growth and development during your baby's first year. He will never change at such a rapid rate again. It is a very important time and a very exciting time as you get to know this very special little person who will share your life.

WEIGHT GAIN:

Shortly after birth your baby will begin gaining about four to seven ounces of weight each week.[1] A general monthly average is anywhere from one to one and a half pounds a month. Of course, babies come in all shapes and sizes, but by the first birthday the typical child will have tripled his/her birth weight and is twenty-eight to thirty-two inches (seventy-one to eighty-one cm) tall.[2]

MILESTONES:

The following chart[3] will give you some general milestones to look for at each stage of development. Although each baby is unique, they follow a similar pattern. The guidelines are approximate. Your baby may reach them a little earlier or a little later and still be in the normal range. If you notice that your baby is behind in several areas at a time, consult with your doctor or a child development specialist.

Birth:

> Sleeps sixteen to eighteen hours a day
> Tightly fisted hands
> Appears to be scrunched or curled up
> Likes to be swaddled
> Eyesight is fuzzy
> Is sensitive to light
> Many movements result from reflexes

SHERRY KELLY

One Month:

Lifts head briefly while lying on stomach
Looks at faces briefly
Watches an object in line of vision
Reduces activity when talked to
Movements still result from reflexes

Two Months:

Lifts head with greater ease
Makes little vocal sounds
Watches and follows moving person
Smiles

Three Months:

Hands are more open and relaxed
Puts hands together
Looks at own hand
Squeals
Laughs

Four Months:

Lifts head and chest when lying on stomach
Rolls over from stomach to back
Puts toys in mouth

Five Months:

Rolls over from back to stomach
Turns head to voice

Reaches for object
Bounces when held in standing position

Six Months:

Sits with help
"Talks" to toys
Eats a cracker
Begins to use cup
Drops things on purpose

Seven Months:

Imitates speech sounds
Tries to put foot in mouth
Eats solid food with spoon
Picks things up
Likes to bang objects on hard surface
Rocks on hands and knees
Passes object from one hand to the other

Eight Months:

Increased shyness with strangers
Plays peek-a-boo
Says "Mama" and "Dada" but not specifically
Holds a toy in each hand at the same time
Responds to name or "hi"

Nine Months:

Sits without support
Bangs two toys together

Can grasp a piece of cereal with thumb and
index finger
Pulls self to standing but does not know how
to get down
Starts to creep or crawl

Ten Months:

Explores and pokes things with fingers
Can change positions from lying down to
sitting up
Plays patty-cake
Walks while holding on to a support
Crawls
Jabbers

Eleven Months:

Says "Mama" and "Dada" with specific meaning
Can pick up tiny things
Can stand alone briefly
Drinks from a cup
Waves "bye-bye"

Twelve Months:

Says "Dada" or "Mama" plus two other words
Takes first steps and begins to walk
Understands simple phrases like "Give it to me"
Stoops and stands again
Walks with one hand held
Plays with ball
Imitates activities (rocking a doll, pushing a car)

OBJECT PERMANENCE:

Object permanence is the ability to know something exists even when it is no longer within sight. It is a less noticed milestone because many parents do not know to look for it. You can test this in your baby by showing him a soft object and then dropping it out of his line of vision. Does he look to see where it has gone? Another way to test this is showing him a toy and then covering it up with a blanket. Does he look for it, or is it "out of sight, out of mind"? If you begin playing this type of game with your baby at about four months, you should see a definite "out of sight, out of mind" reaction. Try it every couple of weeks or so. You can encourage your baby's learning of object permanence by covering up only half of the object.

By about six to eight months, most babies' brains have developed to the point that they know something or someone still exists even though they can no longer see them. This is when—and why—peek-a-boo becomes so much fun! It also is about this time that your baby may start to cry when you leave his sight. This is the first sign of separation anxiety, when baby learns that he is a separate little being and that mom still exists when he does not see her. All of a sudden he has an "I want my mama!" sort of feeling.[4]

When you need to leave your baby with someone else, it may be tempting to sneak off in order to prevent your baby from crying, but this is not a good idea. Your baby will never know when you are going to up and disappear and he may begin to feel insecure. It is best to always tell your baby when you leave (if he is awake), but do not prolong the goodbye when he cries. Just remain calm, give him a quick kiss, tell him you will be back, and then leave.

HELPING YOUR BABY LEARN:

There are many ways you can help your baby learn. As you go about your daily routine, talk to him about what you are doing. Tell him the name of objects you come into contact with. Show him toys and how to play with them. Imitate his vocalizations and actions. Read to him from the very beginning. As he grows, point to pictures in a book and name them and tell him the sounds the animals make, etc. Sing to him all the little children's songs that you know. Play all types of music for him. Quietly playing classical music is thought to help encourage brain development.[5]

Your baby's brain will be developing at an amazing rate. By providing a loving, stimulating, encouraging, and safe environment, you will have a powerful influence on your baby's brain development. A word of caution here: over stimulating and over orchestrating the learning process is unnecessary and can be harmful. Most parents care for their infant in a natural and nurturing way by just being aware of his needs and the things that bring him pleasure. Pay attention to your baby and react accordingly when he lets you know that he is having fun or is tired or wants a more restful activity.[6]

TEETH:

At around three to four months of age, your baby's salivary glands begin to mature and produce more saliva. Because your baby does not know what to do with this extra saliva, drooling may begin. Parents usually think that the drooling means their baby is cutting his first tooth, however, this is not always the case.[7] Most first teeth arrive between the age of five and seven months, but anywhere between birth and eighteen months is considered normal. Generally, babies will have four teeth by their first birthday. The usual pattern is that the two bottom central incisors come in first, followed by the two uppers.[8]

Teething can be uncomfortable for your baby. He may be irritable and fussy for a few days and may not sleep or eat as well. Besides the pain involved when new teeth erupt through tender gums, consider how it must feel to suddenly have a first tooth sticking out in your mouth! To help soothe your baby's irritated gums, provide him with a cool teething ring or a clean washcloth to chew on. Ask your pediatrician before applying a teething gel or giving your baby pain medication.

As soon as the first tooth makes an appearance, begin dental hygiene by using a piece of gauze or a soft cloth and water to clean the tooth and gums. Because babies will swallow it, toothpaste is not recommended until about the age of two years.

Note of caution: If your baby has a fever, diarrhea, or a rash, you should consult your doctor. Many parents overlook a real illness when their baby is teething because they think the symptoms are caused by teething.

DAMAGE CONTROL

SETTING LIMITS:

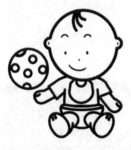

As your baby grows and becomes more independent, it will be necessary to set limits in which he can have the freedom he needs to grow and flourish while his behavior remains acceptable and safe. You can do this by baby proofing your home and simply moving your baby away from items and areas that would be unsafe or inappropriate. Use positive words and phrases as much as possible. For example: "Come away." "That is just to look at." "Come play with your ball." "That is Daddy's camera." "Let's put Grandma's purse on the cabinet." Get into the habit of telling your baby what *to* do rather than just always what *not* to do. Instead of saying, "Don't be mean to the cat!" say, "Pet the cat gently like this."

A very important part of the learning process involves your baby exploring anything and everything that he can get his hands on. It is our responsibility as adults to create an environment that allows baby the opportunity he needs to explore in a safe and acceptable way. You can provide some fun things that are okay for your baby to get into. Clean out a drawer or cabinet in the kitchen and put only safe items like plastic bowls, plastic measuring spoons, and empty spice bottles, etc. back in and give baby your okay to explore. The off-limits drawers and cabinets should be fitted with child-proof latches. Also, fill a box, basket, or other container with toys, sturdy cards, empty shampoo bottles, coasters, etc. and hide it under a table or in a corner for your baby to find.

There are some things that cannot conveniently be put out of reach like stoves, lamps, fireplaces, sharp corners of brick, furniture, etc. Do as much as possible to make these areas safe, and then use words like "hot," "danger," "no-no," etc., keeping a firm tone of voice. Do not confuse your baby by laughing about something he should not be doing. Be consistent and always move baby away from these areas.

Often giving him a toy or other item of interest will distract him for a while. If he continues to approach something that is off-limits, place him in a different room or put him in a playpen or other safe place for a while. Never spank your baby's hand for doing what his curiosity leads him to do. Getting into things is not misbehavior; it is simply what babies this age do—explore and learn about their world. After a while, he will outgrow this stage and move on to the next.

ENCOURAGING GOOD BEHAVIOR:

Busy parents often ignore their little ones when they are being "good" or playing quietly. You may be using these moments to finish something that needs done or to take a minute for yourself. However, this can lead to your baby "acting out" in order to get your attention. To prevent this from happening, notice these quiet times and tell your baby, "I like the way you are playing with your blocks!" and take a minute to play with him. Give your baby a little praise and attention when he is doing something that pleases you, and he will want to do more of this type of activity. Get into the practice of focusing your praise on his behavior instead of saying something about his being a good boy. This early praise will help him feel good about himself and his accomplishments. It will give him the self-esteem he needs to try new things with confidence and begin a pattern of success that can continue throughout his life.

SHERRY KELLY

Keep in mind that your baby will imitate the things he sees and hears. If he is hit or he witnesses hitting, he will do the same. If he hears bad words, he will soon be saying them. The more you can protect him from seeing and hearing undesirable behavior, the easier things will be for all of you. It is imperative that you monitor television programs and movies in his presence. As Benjamin Franklin is often quoted, "An ounce of prevention is worth a pound of cure." [1]

On the other hand, your child will also imitate positive things he sees and hears. Use manners with and around your baby. Say "please" and "thank you." Talk respectfully to him and to others. Let him witness "little acts of kindness."

EXTENDED WARRANTY

KEEP A RECORD:

The first year is a time of rapid change for your baby and your newly established family. One of the most rewarding aspects of being a parent is to share the experiences of learning, growing, and changing from day to day. Enjoy watching your baby. Take pictures to keep and to share. Buy a calendar and make notes of all the "firsts" your baby will accomplish this year. Also keep a record of all your baby's medical visits, including his height and weight.

WHERE TO GET HELP:

If you have questions that were not covered in this material, please ask your pediatrician or other child development specialist. There also is an abundant amount of information available in books and on the Internet—some of it excellent, some not so good. Just because it is there to read does not mean it is accurate. Always look to see where the information is coming from and check different sources to see if they agree. Check the date of publication to see if you have the latest research, as new knowledge puts a new light on things.

ONGOING SUPPORT:

You and your infant are just beginning your life together as a family. New babies grow and change very quickly. *Continue* to educate yourself about child development and each stage of life your child enters. Stay a step ahead. Take a class or read about the next stage as your child reaches it. That way you will be prepared to be an effective parent while guiding your child along his continuing journey.

Ideas:

Think about what family traditions you want to continue with your child. What memories from your childhood do you hold dear? Have you heard of any traditions other families practice that you might like to begin with your baby?

SPIRITUAL GUIDANCE:

Last and most importantly, pray with and for your baby. Pray for God's guidance in raising this precious child you have been entrusted with. We all want our children to have a good life. However, some parents neglect the most important area of growth. To be responsible parents, we must care for our children physically, emotionally, intellectually, and spiritually.

Teaching your child to have faith in God is the best gift you can give. Jesus loves you and your baby and wants the best for you in this life and for all eternity. If you were not raised in a religious home, you can learn along with your child. You might be surprised to know that many young parents first begin to attend church for the sake of their children.

To help your child grow spiritually:

- Begin early

- Read Bible stories

- Take your child to church

- Model appropriate behavior

- Sing "Jesus Loves Me"

- Teach your child to pray

- Look for opportunities to talk to your child about God

- Teach your child to live by "The Golden Rule":

Treat others just as you want to be treated.
Luke 6:31[1]

Happy parenting!

INDEX

REFERENCES

Preliminary Instructions

1   Pregnancy-Info.net, 2001–2008: Cord Blood Banking FAQ, http://www.pregnancy-info.net/cord_blood.html (accessed March 11, 2008)

Important Notice

Setting Up

1   Sherry Kelly, "Preparing Your Nest! (Getting Ready for Baby)" (Canadian County OSU Cooperative Extension Service Home Visitation Program 1992)

2   Jamie Schaefer-Wilson et al., Consumer Reports *Guide to Childproofing & Safety* (New York: Consumers Union of United States, Inc., 2008), 194

3   NHTSA: Child Safety Seat Inspection Stations, http://www.nhtsa.dot.gov/cps/cpsfitting/FindFitting.cfm (accessed June 4, 2008)

4   SAFE KIDS:4 out of 5 Car Seats Are Used Wrong., National SAFE KIDS Campaign Brochure, January, 2000, back.

Registration

1   Bruce Lansky, *The New Baby Name Survey* (Minnetonka : Meadowbrook Press, 2007)ix, x, xi

2   USLEGAL,"Oklahoma Paternity Forms, Documents and Law" http://www.uslegalforms.com/paternity/oklhoma-paternity-forms.htm (accessed March 8, 2008)

3   Sherry Kelly, "Name Me, I'm Yours! (Before Naming Your Baby)" (Canadian County OSU Cooperative Extension Service Home Visitation Program 1992)

Preset Menu

1   Sherry Kelly, "Ready or Not, Here I Come! (What Your Newborn Will Be Like)" (Canadian County OSU Cooperative Extension Service, Home Visitation Program 1992)

2   Shelov, Sreven P., and Robert E. Hannemann, eds., The American Academy of Pediatrics *Caring For Your Baby and Young Child* (New York: Bantam Books, 2005)145–147

System Diagram

1   Steven P. Shelov and Robert E. Hannemann, The American Academy of Pediatrics *Caring For Your Baby and Young Child* (New York: Bantam Books, 2005)36–37

2   Jo Frost, *Confident Baby Care* (New York: Hyperion, 2008) 103

3   The Parenting Group, 2008: Your Baby's Sense of Smell, http://www.parenting.com/article/Baby/Care/Your-Baby's-Sense-of-Smell (accessed September 12, 2008)

4   T. Berry Brazelton, *touchpoints* (Reading: Addison-Wesley Publishing Company, 1992)34–35

5   Steven P. Shelov and Robert E. Hannemann, The American Academy of Pediatrics *Caring For Your Baby and Young Child* (New York: Bantam Books, 2005)154

6   Ibid. 56

7   Sherry Kelly, Ready or Not, Here I come! (What Your Newborn Will Be Like), (Canadian County OSU Cooperative Extension Service Home Visitation Program 1992)

8   Steven P. Shelov and Robert E. Hannemann, The American Academy of Pediatrics *Caring For Your Baby and Young Child* (New York: Bantam Books, 2005)38, 139

9   Sherry Kelly, Ready or Not, Here I come! (What Your Newborn Will Be Like), (Canadian County OSU Cooperative Extension Service Home Visitation Program 1992)

10 Steven P. Shelov and Robert E. Hannemann, The American Academy of Pediatrics *Caring For Your Baby and Young Child* (New York: Bantam Books, 2005)45–47

Some Assembly May Be Required

1   Steven P. Shelov and Robert E. Hannemann, The American Academy of Pediatrics *Caring For Your Baby and Young Child* (New York: Bantam Books, 2005)13–15

2   Ibid.

Installation

1   Sherry Kelly, We've Only Just Begun! (Time of Adjustment), (Canadian County OSU Cooperative Extension Service Home Visitation Program 1992)

Power On

1   Harvey Karp, *The Happiest Baby on the Block* (New York: Bantam Books, Paper Back 2003)126–127

2   Mary D. Salter Ainsworth and John Bowlby, "American Psychologist." Vol. 46 (4) April 1991, 333–341.

3   Sherry Kelly, The World Is Okay! (How Baby Learns To Trust), (Canadian County OSU Cooperative Extension Service Home Visitation Program 1992)

Maintenance

1   Erik Lykke Mortensen, PhD, et al., "The Association Between Duration of Breastfeeding and Adult Intelligence," The Journal of the American Medical Association, May 8, 2002, Vol. 287 No. 18

2   New Jersey WIC Breastfeeding Services, "Benefits of Breastfeeding," Trenton, NJ, November 15, 2005

3   La Leche League, "Breastfeeding...The Best Beginning," Beaverton, Oregon, October 26, 2007

4   Jamie Eloise Bolane and Karen Martin Tomaselli, "Breastfeeding Getting Started in 5 Easy Steps" Brochure, (Childbirth Graphics, Waco, TX)

5   Linda Murray et al., *the babycenter essential guide to your baby's first year* (New York: Rodale Inc., 2007)81

6   La Leche League International: Find a La Leche League Leader or Group Near You in the USA, 2008, http:www.llli.org/WebUS.html (accessed August 13, 2008)

7   Sherry Kelly, One To Grow On! (Breastfeeding), (Canadian County OSU Cooperative Extension Service Home Visitaion Program 1992)

8   Lisa A. Flam, "Worried parents returning to use of glass baby bottles," *The Oklahoman*, March 30, 2008, Living section 5D.

9   The Associated Press, "Chemical is not dangerous, FDA says," *The Oklahoman*, August 16, 2008, Business section 3B.

10 Steven P. Shelov and Robert E. Hannemann, The American Academy of Pediatrics *Caring For Your Baby and Young Child* (New York: Bantam Books, 2005) 113

11 Ibid.

12 Ibid. 107

13 Steven P. Shelov and Robert E. Hannemann, The American Academy of Pediatrics *Caring For Your Baby and Young Child* (New York: Bantam Books, 2005)33, 141

14 Ibid. 57–60

15 Linda Murray et al., *the babycenter essential guide to your baby's first year* (New York: Rodale Inc., 2007)108–109

16 Laura Walther Nathanson, *The Portable Pediatrician For Parents* (New York: HarperPerennial, 1982)65

17 DeCare International, "A Baby's First Tooth" (Minnesota, 2006)

18   Jo Frost, *Confident Baby Care* (New York: Hyperion, 2008)131

19   American Academy of Pediatrics: Choking Prevention, 2/07, http://www.aap.org/publiced/br-choking.htm (accessed September 2, 2008)

Noise Reduction

1   Parenting iVillage.com, 1995–2008: The Newborn's Six States of Consciousness http://parenting.ivillage.com/newborn/0,,lz_6qvd,00.html (accessed February 23, 2008)

Operating Precautions

1   Catherine Roca, Depression During and After Pregnancy (National Women's Health Information Center, April 2005)1–5

Safety Precautions

1   Anne H. Soukhanov, Sen. Ed. Et al., *Webster's 2 New Riverside University Dictionary* (Boston:Houghton Mifflin Company, 1984)1030

2   Jamie Schaefer-Wilson et al., Consumer Reports *Guide to Childproofing & Safety* (New York:Consumers Union of United States, Inc., 2008)5, 67

3   Public Awareness Campaign, Never Shake a Baby! (Oklahoma Committee for Prevention of Child Abuse, Oklahoma State Department of Health)

4   Jamie Schaefer-Wilson et al., Consumer Reports
     Guide to Childproofing & Safety (New York:Con-
     sumers Union of United States, Inc., 2008)9

5   OSF HealthCare: Healthsteps Lead Paint Warn-
     ing, http://www.stayinginshape.com/3osfcorp/libv/
     k10.shtml (accessed August 16, 2008)

Trouble Shooting

1   Steven P. Shelov and Robert E. Hannemann, The
     American Academy of Pediatrics *Caring For Your
     Baby and Young Child* (New York: Bantam Books,
     2005)67

Limited Warranty

1   Linda Murray et al., *the babycenter essential guide
     to your baby's first year* (New York: Rodale Inc.,
     2007)110

2   Steven P. Shelov and Robert E. Hannemann, The
     American Academy of Pediatrics *Caring For Your
     Baby and Young Child* (New York: Bantam Books,
     2005)232

3   TPT, Birth to One Year: Developmental Mile-
     stones. 224

4   T. Berry Brazelton, *touchpoints* (Reading: Addison-
     Wesley Publishing Company, 1992)114–116

5   Diane Bales, Building Baby's Brain: The Role of Music, 2003–2008, http://www.educationoasis.com/resources/Articles/building_babys_brain.htm (accessed August 8, 2008)

6   Kathryn Vaughn, Wired for Learning: Promoting Infant Brain Development, http://www.forever-families.net/xml/articles/infant_brain_devt.aspx (accessed February 29, 2008)

7   Riley Hospital for Children, Birth to 6 Months, Baby Teeth, http://rileychildrenshospital.com/parents-and-patients/caring-for-kids/birthto6month-schpt2.jsp (accessed March 8, 2008)

8   Theodosia Sideropoulos Spewock, *A Year of Fun Just for Babies,* The 8-Month-Old, (Everett: Totline Books, 1995)

Damage Control

1   Ushistory.org. The electric BEN FRANKLIN, http://www.ushistory.org/franklin/quotable/quote67.htm (accessed August 13, 2008)

Extended Warranty

1   American Bible Society, *The HOLY BIBLE* Contemporary English Version (New York, 1995), 1064

Author Sherry Kelly is devoted to God and family, and she has always held a special love for children. While raising their family, Sherry and her husband took care of foster babies. This firsthand experience with broken families encouraged her desire to help future parents gain the knowledge they need to succeed. When her own three children were young adults, she went to college and later became a parent educator. As a family support worker with the Healthy Families program, Sherry made visits to the homes of young mothers to teach them effective parenting skills. Now her book of instructions will help other moms and dads as they enter the exciting world of parenthood.

Sherry and her husband, Don, live in Yukon, Oklahoma. They have three adult children and eight grandchildren.